Fascial Exercise Made Easy

Understanding the Fascial System

By

Eilidh Fergus

Copyright@2023

Table of Contents

CHAPTER 1

Introduction

1.1 What is Fascial Exercise?

Fascial exercise, also known as fascial fitness or fascial training, is a specialized approach to physical fitness and wellness that focuses on the health and flexibility of the fascial system in the human body. The fascia is a complex network of connective tissue that wraps around and permeates every muscle, bone, organ, and even individual cells. It plays a pivotal role in maintaining the structural integrity of the body, transmitting force, and facilitating movement. Fascial exercise involves a range of techniques and movements specifically designed to target and improve the condition of the fascial network.

Fascial exercise differs from traditional muscle-centric exercise because it acknowledges the importance of the entire fascial system. While traditional strength training and aerobic exercise primarily target muscle development, fascial exercise emphasizes the holistic approach of strengthening and mobilizing not just the muscles but also the fascial tissues that connect and envelop them. These exercises can include various movements, stretches, and self-myofascial release techniques that aim to optimize the function and health of the fascia.

1.2 Importance of Fascia in the Body

Understanding the significance of the fascial system in the body is crucial to appreciate the value of fascial exercise. The fascia serves as a comprehensive connective web that maintains the structural integrity of the body. It can be divided into three primary layers:

Superficial Fascia:

This layer lies just beneath the skin and contains fat and blood vessels. It helps to store and distribute energy, acts as an insulator, and provides a protective cushion for underlying structures.

Deep Fascia:

Deep fascia envelops muscles and groups of muscles. It assists in creating compartments within the body, allowing muscles to glide smoothly against one another. It also transmits mechanical forces generated during movement.

Visceral Fascia:

This layer surrounds the internal organs, providing support, protection, and helping to maintain the position of organs within the body.

The fascial system is essential for several reasons:

1. **Structural Support**: It ensures the body's stability and alignment by connecting and holding muscles, bones, and organs in their proper places.

2. **Force Transmission**: Fascia is involved in transmitting mechanical forces generated by

muscle contractions, which is critical for efficient and coordinated movement.

3. **Injury Prevention**: Healthy fascia can help prevent injuries by maintaining the body's structural balance and supporting joints and muscles.

4. **Pain Management**: Tight or restricted fascia can lead to pain and discomfort. Properly conditioned fascia can reduce or eliminate chronic pain and improve overall comfort.

5. **Optimized Performance**: For athletes and fitness enthusiasts, healthy fascia can lead to improved performance by enhancing flexibility, mobility, and strength.

6. **Overall Well-being**: A balanced and well-maintained fascial system contributes to general well-being, vitality, and a sense of lightness in the body.

1.3 Benefits of Fascial Exercise

Fascial exercise offers a multitude of benefits that extend beyond conventional exercise routines. Here are some of the advantages:

1. Enhanced Flexibility and Range of Motion:

Fascial exercises target the fascial tissues, which, when healthy and supple, improve joint mobility and flexibility. This can be particularly beneficial for athletes, dancers, and anyone looking to increase their range of motion.

2. Improved Posture:

By addressing the deep fascia that supports the body's structure, fascial exercise helps correct postural imbalances and can alleviate issues related to poor posture, such as back and neck pain.

3. Pain Reduction and Management:

For individuals suffering from chronic pain conditions, fascial exercise can be a non-invasive and effective approach to alleviate pain by releasing tension and promoting tissue health.

4. Injury Prevention:

Healthy fascia reduces the risk of injury by maintaining proper biomechanics and supporting the musculoskeletal system. This is particularly important for athletes and individuals engaged in physical activities.

5. Stress Reduction:

Fascial exercise often involves mindful movement and deep breathing, which can help reduce stress and promote relaxation. This mind-body connection is an integral part of fascial exercise routines.

6. Holistic Wellness:

Fascial exercise promotes a holistic approach to wellness by considering the interconnectedness of the body's various systems. It encourages a sense of balance and harmony, not only physically but also mentally and emotionally.

fascial exercise is a holistic approach to physical fitness that recognizes the vital role of the fascial system in the body. It offers numerous benefits, including enhanced flexibility, improved posture, pain reduction, injury prevention, stress reduction, and overall well-being. Understanding the importance of fascia in the body is fundamental to appreciating the value of these specialized exercise routines.

CHAPTER 2

Understanding the Fascial System

2.1 Anatomy of Fascia

Fascia is a complex and pervasive connective tissue that plays a fundamental role in the structural integrity and functioning of the human body. To understand the importance of fascial exercise, it's essential to grasp the basic anatomy of fascia. Fascia can be divided into various layers, each with distinct characteristics and functions:

Superficial Fascia:

- **Location**: This layer is situated just beneath the skin and covers the entire body.

- **Composition**: Superficial fascia is primarily composed of adipose tissue (fat) and loose connective tissue.

- **Functions**: It acts as an insulator, providing thermal regulation, and functions as a storage site for energy. It also contains blood vessels and nerves and plays a role in proprioception (the body's awareness of its position in space).

Deep Fascia:

- **Location**: Deep fascia is found deeper within the body, surrounding muscles and muscle groups.

- **Composition**: It is made up of denser connective tissue, including collagen and elastin fibers.

- **Functions**: Deep fascia creates compartments within the body, enveloping muscle groups and allowing them to move smoothly against one another. It provides support and protection for muscles and facilitates the transmission of mechanical forces generated during movement.

Visceral Fascia:

- **Location**: Visceral fascia surrounds internal organs within the body.

- **Composition**: It consists of layers of connective tissue that provide a protective sheath around organs.

- **Functions**: Visceral fascia offers support and stability to organs, enabling them to maintain their position and function correctly.

Perineural Fascia:

- **Location**: This specialized type of fascia surrounds nerves in the body.

- **Composition**: It contains collagen fibers and is integral to the health and function of nerves.

- **Functions**: Perineural fascia provides protection and support for nerves, allowing them to transmit electrical signals efficiently.

**Endomysium, Perimysium, and
Epimysium:**

- **Location**: These types of fascia
  are specific to muscle tissue.

- **Composition**: They consist of
  collagen fibers.

- **Functions**: Endomysium
  surrounds individual muscle
  fibers, perimysium surrounds
  bundles of muscle fibers
  (fascicles), and epimysium
  envelops entire muscles. They
  provide support and structure to
  muscles, enabling them to
  contract effectively.

Understanding the anatomy of fascia
is crucial for appreciating its role in
maintaining the body's structural
integrity and facilitating movement.
This knowledge forms the basis for

the development and practice of
fascial exercise techniques.

2.2 Types of Fascia

Fascia can be categorized into
different types based on its location
and function within the body. These
distinct types of fascia play various
roles in ensuring the body's
functionality and structural support.
Here are the primary types of fascia:

1. Superficial Fascia:

- **Location**: Found just beneath
  the skin.

- **Function**: Superficial fascia
  serves as an insulator, energy
  storage, and contains blood
  vessels and nerves.

2. Deep Fascia:

- **Location**: Surrounds muscles and muscle groups.

- **Function**: Provides structural support for muscles, allowing them to function together efficiently. It also transmits forces generated during movement.

3. Visceral Fascia:

- **Location**: Envelopes and supports internal organs within the body.

- **Function**: Ensures the proper position and functioning of organs by providing a protective sheath.

4. Perineural Fascia:

- **Location**: Surrounds nerves in the body.

- **Function**: Protects and supports nerves, aiding in the efficient transmission of electrical signals.

5. Endomysium, Perimysium, and Epimysium:

- **Location**: Specific to muscle tissue.

- **Function**: These types of fascia provide support and structure to muscles, allowing them to contract effectively and transmit forces during movement.

Understanding these types of fascia and their distinct functions is crucial for comprehending how fascial exercise can target and benefit different aspects of the fascial system, ultimately improving the body's overall health and performance.

Fascial exercise techniques are designed to optimize the condition of these various types of fascia, leading to increased flexibility, reduced pain, and enhanced well-being.

2.3 Functions of Fascia

Fascia is a versatile and interconnected web of connective tissue that serves a range of crucial functions in the human body. Understanding these functions is essential for appreciating the significance of fascial exercise and its impact on overall health and well-being. Here are the primary functions of fascia:

1. **Structural Integrity**: Fascia plays a pivotal role in maintaining the structural integrity of the body. It wraps

around and permeates every muscle, bone, organ, and even individual cells. By connecting and holding these structures in their proper places, fascia provides stability and support.

2. **Force Transmission**: Fascia is involved in the transmission of mechanical forces generated by muscle contractions. When you move, your muscles contract and exert force on your bones and other tissues. The fascial system ensures that these forces are effectively distributed and transmitted throughout the body.

3. **Biomechanical Efficiency**: Fascia facilitates efficient biomechanics by enabling muscles to glide smoothly against one another. This is

essential for coordinated and fluid movement. Healthy fascia minimizes friction and ensures that muscles work together harmoniously.

4. **Joint Stabilization**: Fascia contributes to joint stability by supporting the ligaments and tendons that connect bones and muscles. Strong, well-conditioned fascia helps prevent excessive joint mobility and reduces the risk of injuries.

5. **Protection and Cushioning**: Superficial fascia, located just beneath the skin, acts as a protective cushion for underlying structures. It provides a layer of insulation and guards against external trauma.

6. **Energy Storage**: The superficial fascia contains adipose tissue (fat), which serves as an energy store. This stored energy can be mobilized when needed for activities like exercise or to maintain body temperature.

7. **Proprioception**: Fascia contains a network of sensory receptors that contribute to proprioception, which is the body's ability to sense its position in space. These receptors provide feedback to the nervous system, helping to maintain balance and coordination.

8. **Pain Regulation**: In cases of injury or chronic conditions, fascia can become tight or restricted, leading to pain and

discomfort. By releasing tension and restrictions in fascia through methods like myofascial release, pain can be reduced or alleviated.

9. **Improved Circulation**: Fascial release techniques can help improve blood and lymphatic circulation, which can have a positive impact on tissue health and overall well-being.

10. **Facilitation of Movement**: Fascia ensures that muscles and other soft tissues can move freely without constraints. It supports the range of motion and flexibility necessary for activities of daily living and physical performance.

11. **Overall Well-being**: A balanced and well-maintained

fascial system contributes to a sense of well-being, vitality, and a feeling of lightness in the body. It can help reduce physical and mental tension.

Understanding these functions of fascia underscores the importance of fascial exercise in maintaining and enhancing the health and performance of the fascial system. Through specific techniques and movements, fascial exercise aims to optimize these functions, resulting in improved flexibility, reduced pain, and a greater sense of physical and mental well-being.

CHAPTER 3

Principles of Fascial Exercise

Fascial exercise is a holistic approach to physical fitness and wellness that incorporates a unique set of principles to optimize the health and function of the fascial system.

3.1 Mind-Body Connection

The mind-body connection is a core principle of fascial exercise that emphasizes the integration of mental awareness and intention with physical movement. This principle recognizes that the mind and body are intricately linked, and the quality of movement is greatly influenced by one's mental focus. Here's a closer look at the role of the mind-body connection in fascial exercise:

- **Awareness**: Practitioners of fascial exercise are encouraged to develop a heightened sense of body awareness. This involves paying close attention to how the body feels during movements, identifying areas of tension or discomfort, and recognizing the impact of specific movements on the fascial system.

- **Conscious Movement**: Mindful and intentional movement is a cornerstone of fascial exercise. Instead of going through the motions mechanically, individuals are encouraged to consciously engage with their bodies, focusing on the subtleties of movement and alignment.

- **Breath Control**: The breath is a powerful tool for establishing a mind-body connection. Proper breathing techniques are integrated into fascial exercise routines to enhance relaxation, reduce tension, and support fluid movement. Breath awareness helps individuals synchronize their breath with movement.

- **Release of Tension**: By bringing awareness to areas of tension and discomfort, individuals can use the mind-body connection to release fascial restrictions. Mindful breathing and visualization techniques can be used to encourage the fascia to relax and unwind, leading to improved flexibility and reduced pain.

- **Stress Reduction**: The mind-body connection in fascial exercise can be a source of stress reduction. As individuals focus on the present moment and their physical sensations, they can experience relaxation and relief from stress and anxiety.

- **Integration with Other Practices**: Many fascial exercise methods, such as yoga and Pilates, incorporate the mind-body connection as a central component of their practice. These practices encourage a holistic approach to health and wellness.

The mind-body connection in fascial exercise is not limited to the physical aspect of movement but extends to emotional and mental well-being. It promotes a sense of balance, presence, and a deeper understanding of one's body, which can have profound benefits for overall health.

3.2 Dynamic Movements

Dynamic movements are another fundamental principle of fascial exercise. These movements are designed to engage the fascial system by encouraging multi-dimensional and varied motion patterns. Dynamic movements differ from traditional exercises that focus solely on muscle-centric, linear motions. Here's why dynamic movements are integral to fascial exercise:

- **Multi-Planar Motion**: Dynamic movements involve motion in multiple planes and directions. Rather than just moving forward and backward, dynamic exercises incorporate side-to-side, rotational, and diagonal movements. This challenges the fascial system in diverse ways, promoting flexibility and adaptability.

- **Stretch and Recoil**: Dynamic movements often include movements that stretch the fascia and allow it to recoil. This stretching and releasing action is particularly beneficial for fascial health. It encourages the fascia to regain elasticity and maintain optimal hydration.

- **Full-Body Integration**:
  Dynamic movements engage
  the entire body, from head to
  toe. They promote a sense of
  wholeness and
  interconnectedness within the
  body, emphasizing that the
  fascial system connects all
  regions of the body and plays a
  role in every movement.

- **Functional Fitness**: Dynamic
  movements mimic real-life
  functional activities, which are
  multi-dimensional and dynamic
  in nature. This makes fascial
  exercise highly relevant to
  everyday movements and
  activities, enhancing overall
  fitness and performance.

- **Balance and Coordination**:
  Dynamic movements challenge
  balance and coordination as

they require the body to adapt to varying movement patterns. This enhances proprioception and spatial awareness.

- **Injury Prevention**: By engaging the fascial system through dynamic movements, individuals can reduce the risk of injury by improving joint stability, enhancing flexibility, and maintaining proper biomechanics.

- **Holistic Approach**: Dynamic movements align with the holistic approach of fascial exercise, as they target not only muscle groups but also the fascial tissues that envelop and connect them.

Incorporating dynamic movements into a fascial exercise routine ensures that the fascial system is stimulated comprehensively, leading to improved flexibility, reduced tension, and a heightened sense of physical vitality. These movements are a key component of various fascial exercise methods and contribute to the holistic well-being of practitioners.

3.3 Breath and Fascial Exercise

Breath control is a fundamental and distinctive aspect of fascial exercise. The breath is intimately connected to the fascial system and plays a critical role in optimizing the health and function of fascia. This principle, often referred to as "breathwork" or "breath awareness," is an integral part of fascial exercise for several reasons:

1. Facilitating Relaxation

The breath is a powerful tool for promoting relaxation and reducing tension within the fascial system. When individuals focus on their breath during exercise, they can consciously release areas of tension within the fascia. This relaxation can lead to improved flexibility, greater comfort, and reduced pain. Deep, controlled breaths promote a state of calmness, which is conducive to fascial release.

2. Enhancing Mobility

Proper breathing techniques can enhance the mobility of fascia by encouraging the release of restrictions and adhesions within the connective tissue. Deep diaphragmatic breathing, in particular, helps stretch and release the fascia, especially in the chest, ribcage, and abdominal areas. This increased mobility can improve posture, reduce stiffness, and enhance overall movement.

3. Oxygenation of Tissues

Effective breathing ensures that the body receives an adequate supply of oxygen, which is vital for maintaining the health of fascia and other tissues. Oxygen plays a key role in cellular repair and regeneration, helping to maintain the fascial network's integrity and functionality.

4. Mind-Body Connection

Breath awareness fosters a strong mind-body connection, aligning with the core principle of fascial exercise. Individuals become more attuned to their physical sensations, emotional state, and energy levels when they consciously link their breath to movement. This heightened awareness can lead to a more profound understanding of the body's needs and limitations.

5. Stress Reduction

Fascial exercise often incorporates deep, rhythmic breathing patterns, which can act as a stress reduction technique. By focusing on the breath and the present moment, individuals can mitigate the effects of stress and anxiety. Stress reduction is particularly important because chronic stress can contribute to fascial restrictions and discomfort.

6. Support for Movement

The breath can provide support for dynamic movements in fascial exercise routines. By coordinating breath with specific movements, individuals can enhance their performance, maintain proper alignment, and reduce the risk of injury. Breath control helps synchronize the body's actions, ensuring that the fascial system is engaged optimally.

7. Holistic Wellness

The combination of breath, movement, and awareness in fascial exercise aligns with a holistic approach to wellness. It promotes not only physical health but also mental and emotional well-being. The breath is a unifying element that ties together the various facets of holistic wellness, reinforcing the interconnectedness of the mind and body.

The principle of breath in fascial exercise underscores the importance of conscious, controlled breathing during exercise routines. By integrating breath awareness into fascial exercise, individuals can facilitate relaxation, enhance mobility, oxygenate their tissues, strengthen the mind-body connection, reduce stress, support movement, and embrace a holistic approach to overall well-being. Breath control is a foundational element that contributes to the effectiveness and depth of fascial exercise practices.

CHAPTER 4

Fascial Exercise Techniques

Fascial exercise encompasses a variety of specialized techniques designed to optimize the health and function of the fascial system.

4.1 Self-Myofascial Release

Self-myofascial release (SMR), also known as self-massage, is a technique that involves applying pressure to specific areas of the body to release tension and restrictions within the fascial network. SMR is typically performed using various tools, such as foam rollers, massage balls, or other self-massage devices. The goal of SMR is to improve fascial mobility and reduce discomfort. Here's how self-myofascial release works:

- **Targeted Pressure**: SMR focuses on specific areas of the body where fascial restrictions, knots, or adhesions may have formed. By applying targeted pressure to these areas, individuals aim to release tension and restore the fascia's natural elasticity.

- **Improved Circulation**: SMR can enhance blood flow to the targeted areas, which aids in the healing and rejuvenation of fascial tissues. It can also help alleviate pain and discomfort by promoting better circulation.

- **Self-Awareness**: Self-myofascial release encourages individuals to become more attuned to their bodies. By actively participating in the process, they can identify areas of tension and discomfort and tailor their self-massage techniques to address specific issues.

- **Flexibility and Mobility**: Regular self-myofascial release can lead to increased flexibility and improved range of motion. It's especially valuable for athletes, as it can support enhanced athletic performance and help prevent injuries.

- **Stress Reduction**: The practice of self-myofascial release can be calming and stress-reducing. The deep pressure and focused attention on the body can promote relaxation and a sense of well-being.

Tools commonly used in self-myofascial release include foam rollers, lacrosse balls, massage sticks, and specialized self-massage devices designed to target various muscle groups and fascial areas. Practitioners typically apply pressure to specific points along the fascial lines, holding the pressure for a period of time to release tension gradually.

4.2 Fascial Stretching

Fascial stretching is a technique that focuses on elongating and conditioning the fascial system, emphasizing a different approach than traditional static stretching. Fascial stretching targets the entire fascial network, aiming to improve flexibility, reduce discomfort, and optimize movement patterns. Here's how fascial stretching differs from conventional stretching:

- **Multi-Planar Movements**: Fascial stretching incorporates multi-dimensional movements that take into account the interconnectedness of the fascial system. This includes stretches in various planes, such as rotational, diagonal, and spiral motions, to challenge the fascia in different ways.

- **Stretch and Release**: Fascial stretching aims to stretch the fascia and encourage it to regain its natural elasticity. This is done through movements that emphasize the concept of stretching and then releasing, mimicking the fascia's natural behavior.

- **Continuous Flow**: Unlike static stretching, which involves holding a stretch for a set duration, fascial stretching often involves a continuous flow of movement. This dynamic approach keeps the fascia engaged throughout the stretching routine.

- **Whole-Body Integration**: Fascial stretching recognizes the importance of addressing the entire body as a connected unit. Movements are designed to engage multiple muscle groups and fascial lines simultaneously, promoting full-body integration and balance.

- **Proprioception**: Fascial stretching can enhance proprioception (the body's sense of its position in space) by involving complex movement patterns that challenge balance and coordination. This heightened awareness of body position contributes to improved movement and posture.

- **Functional Movements**: Fascial stretching often incorporates movements that mimic functional activities, making it relevant to daily life and athletic performance. It focuses on the quality of movement, not just the range of motion.

Fascial stretching can be performed independently or with the guidance of a trained professional, such as a physical therapist, yoga instructor, or fascial stretch therapist. It is particularly beneficial for individuals seeking to improve their flexibility, reduce discomfort, enhance athletic performance, and maintain a balanced and functional body.

Both self-myofascial release and fascial stretching are integral components of fascial exercise, and they complement one another in promoting fascial health, overall well-being, and improved physical performance. These techniques contribute to the holistic approach to health and fitness within the realm of fascial exercise.

4.3 Fascial Sliding

Fascial sliding is a specialized technique within the realm of fascial exercise that focuses on the dynamic and integrated movements of the fascial system. This technique emphasizes the notion that fascia is a continuous web of connective tissue that envelops and links various parts of the body. Fascial sliding involves coordinated movements that target the entire fascial network, promoting flexibility, improved mobility, and overall fascial health. Here's a closer look at fascial sliding:

- **Integrated Movement**: Fascial sliding prioritizes integrated, multi-planar movements that engage the entire body. These movements are designed to encourage the fascia to glide and stretch smoothly. The fascial system is interconnected, and movements in one part of the body can affect distant regions, which is why integrated, whole-body movements are emphasized.

- **Stretch and Release**: Similar to other fascial exercise techniques, fascial sliding involves the concept of stretch and release. During these movements, the fascia is gently stretched and then allowed to recoil. This stretching and releasing action helps improve the fascia's elasticity and mobility.

- **Multi-Directional**: Fascial sliding incorporates movements in multiple directions, including lateral, diagonal, and rotational motions. These varied

movement patterns challenge
the fascia in diverse ways,
ensuring that it is conditioned
thoroughly.

- **Mindful Practice**: Practitioners
of fascial sliding are
encouraged to maintain
mindfulness throughout the
practice. This includes paying
attention to body sensations,
alignment, and breath.
Mindfulness enhances the
mind-body connection and
optimizes the benefits of fascial
sliding.

- **Balance and Proprioception**:
Fascial sliding often includes
movements that challenge
balance and proprioception. By
moving through complex,
multi-dimensional patterns,
individuals develop a

heightened awareness of their body's position in space. This can improve balance and coordination.

- **Functional Fitness**: Many movements within the fascial sliding technique are functionally relevant. They mimic real-life activities, making this form of exercise valuable for enhancing performance in daily activities, sports, and other physical endeavors.

- **Holistic Approach**: Fascial sliding aligns with the holistic approach of fascial exercise by emphasizing the interconnectedness of the body. It recognizes that the fascial system is integral to every aspect of movement and strives to optimize its functionality for improved overall well-being.

Fascial sliding can be practiced independently or under the guidance of a trained professional, such as a physical therapist or a practitioner of fascial stretch therapy. It is particularly beneficial for individuals looking to enhance their flexibility, mobility, and balance, as well as those interested in a holistic approach to wellness and fitness. By incorporating fascial sliding into their routines, individuals can experience a greater sense of physical vitality and well-being.

CHAPTER 5

Tools and Equipment for Fascial Exercise

Fascial exercise utilizes various tools and equipment to enhance the effectiveness of the techniques and optimize the health of the fascial system.

5.1 Foam Rollers

Foam rollers are cylindrical, foam-covered devices that are an integral part of many fascial exercise routines. These tools are designed to assist with self-myofascial release and fascial stretching. Here's how foam rollers are used in fascial exercise and their benefits:

- **Self-Myofascial Release**: Foam rollers are often employed in self-myofascial release (SMR) techniques. By applying pressure and rolling specific areas of the body over the foam roller, individuals can target and release fascial restrictions, knots, and adhesions. This promotes fascial mobility and reduces discomfort.

- **Improved Circulation**: The pressure applied by foam rollers can enhance blood flow to the areas being targeted. This increased circulation contributes to the healing and rejuvenation of fascial tissues, helping to alleviate pain and improve overall fascial health.

- **Full-Body Engagement**: Foam rollers can be used to address various muscle groups and fascial areas, providing a comprehensive approach to fascial exercise. They engage the fascial system throughout the body and are versatile for use in different exercises.

- **Flexibility and Range of Motion**: Regular use of foam rollers can lead to increased flexibility and improved range of motion. This is particularly valuable for athletes and individuals looking to enhance their athletic performance and prevent injuries.

- **Self-Awareness**: Foam rollers encourage individuals to become more aware of their bodies. By actively participating in self-myofascial release with a foam roller, they can identify areas of tension and discomfort, fostering greater body awareness.

- **Stress Reduction**: The deep pressure and focused attention associated with foam rolling can be calming and stress-reducing. It promotes relaxation and a sense of well-being, making it a valuable tool for holistic health.

Foam rollers are available in various sizes, densities, and surface textures, allowing individuals to choose the one that best suits their needs and comfort levels. They are accessible and can be used by people of different fitness levels, making them a popular choice for fascial exercise.

5.2 Massage Balls

Massage balls are small, firm, often rubber or textured balls used for self-myofascial release and targeted massage in fascial exercise. These balls are specifically designed to apply pressure to localized areas of the body. Here's how massage balls are used and their benefits:

- **Precise Targeting**: Massage balls are excellent for pinpointing specific areas of tension, knots, or adhesions in the fascial network. Their small size and focused pressure allow for precise targeting of these problematic spots.

- **Deep Tissue Release**: Massage balls provide deep tissue massage, which can effectively release fascial restrictions and alleviate discomfort. The firmness and texture of the balls enable them to reach deep layers of the fascia.

- **Versatile Use**: Massage balls can be used on various body parts, such as the feet, back, shoulders, hips, and legs. They are versatile tools for self-myofascial release and can complement other fascial exercise techniques.

- **Portability**: Massage balls are portable and easy to carry, making them suitable for use at home, in the gym, or while traveling. Their compact size allows for on-the-go fascial release.

- **Enhanced Circulation**: Similar to foam rollers, massage balls can enhance blood flow to the targeted areas, which promotes tissue health and supports pain relief.

- **Stress Reduction**: The process of using massage balls for self-myofascial release can be relaxing and help reduce stress. It encourages a sense of relaxation and well-being.

Massage balls are available in different sizes and textures to accommodate varying preferences and needs. They are particularly beneficial for individuals seeking a more localized and intense approach to fascial exercise and self-myofascial release.

5.3 Stretching Bands

Stretching bands, also commonly known as resistance bands or exercise bands, are versatile tools that play a valuable role in fascial exercise routines. These bands are made of flexible, elastic material and can be utilized to enhance stretching, strength training, and mobility exercises. Here's how stretching bands are used in fascial exercise and their benefits:

- **Enhanced Stretching**: Stretching bands add resistance to traditional stretches, making them more effective at targeting fascial restrictions. By incorporating resistance into stretches, individuals can stretch the fascial tissues more deeply, promoting better flexibility and mobility.

- **Full-Body Engagement**: Stretching bands allow for a holistic approach to fascial exercise by engaging multiple muscle groups and fascial lines. These bands can be used in various exercises to address different parts of the body simultaneously.

- **Progressive Resistance**: Stretching bands come in different resistance levels, from light to heavy. This provides the flexibility to adjust the level of resistance, making them suitable for individuals of all fitness levels. As strength and flexibility improve, individuals can progress to higher resistance bands.

- **Dynamic Movements**: Stretching bands can be used to perform dynamic movements that challenge the fascial system in multi-dimensional ways. These movements can mimic functional activities and improve balance and coordination.

- **Injury Prevention**: Stretching bands can assist in strengthening the muscles and fascial tissues, reducing the risk of injuries. They are commonly used in rehabilitation and physical therapy to aid in the recovery process.

- **Portability**: Stretching bands are lightweight and portable, making them convenient for use at home, in the gym, or during travel. They provide an accessible and versatile means of engaging in fascial exercise.

- **Variety of Exercises**: Stretching bands can be used in a wide range of exercises, including stretching, strength training, mobility exercises, and even some forms of resistance training. This versatility makes them a valuable addition to any fascial exercise routine.

- **Mind-Body Connection**: The use of stretching bands can foster a strong mind-body connection. Individuals must maintain proper form, posture, and tension while using the bands, enhancing body awareness and alignment.

- **Holistic Approach**: Stretching bands align with the holistic approach of fascial exercise by emphasizing the interconnectedness of the body's systems and addressing overall wellness.

Stretching bands come in various shapes and sizes, including looped bands and straight bands with handles. They can be used to facilitate various types of stretches and exercises, making them adaptable for different fascial exercise methods and goals. Stretching bands are a valuable tool for enhancing flexibility, promoting mobility, and optimizing the health of the fascial system.

CHAPTER 6

Sample Fascial Exercise Routines

6.1 Full-Body Fascial Release Routine

A full-body fascial release routine is a comprehensive series of exercises designed to target and release fascial restrictions throughout the entire body. This routine can help improve flexibility, reduce discomfort, and promote a sense of well-being. Here's a sample full-body fascial release routine:

Equipment Needed: Foam roller, massage balls, stretching bands (optional)

Duration: Approximately 20-30 minutes

Warm-up:

- Begin with 5-10 minutes of light aerobic exercise (e.g., brisk walking or jogging) to increase blood flow and prepare the body for fascial release.

1. Foam Rolling for the Back:

- Lie on your back with a foam roller positioned beneath your upper back.

- Support your head with your hands, keeping your neck relaxed.

- Roll slowly up and down the length of your upper back, from the base of your neck to the middle of your back.

- Focus on areas that feel tense or tight, and pause on those spots for 20-30 seconds to allow for release.

2. Massage Ball Release for the Feet:

- Sit on a chair or the floor with a massage ball under one foot.

- Roll the ball under your foot, paying special attention to the arch and the heel.

- Spend 1-2 minutes on each foot.

3. Stretching Bands for Leg and Hip Release (optional):

- Attach a stretching band to a secure anchor point.

- Place the band around your ankle and lie on your back.

- Gently move your leg in different directions to stretch and release the fascia of the leg and hip.

- Repeat with the other leg.

4. Foam Rolling for the IT Band:

- Lie on your side with the foam roller positioned under the side of your leg, near the hip.

- Roll from your hip down to just above the knee.

- Focus on any tight or tender spots, pausing for 20-30 seconds.

5. Massage Ball Release for the Shoulders:

- Stand with your back against a wall.

- Place a massage ball between the wall and your upper back/shoulder area.

- Move your body to target different areas of your shoulders, releasing any tension.

6. Fascial Stretching for the Chest and Arms (optional):

- Use a stretching band to perform arm stretches that target the chest and shoulder fascia.

- These stretches should be held for 20-30 seconds on each side.

7. Foam Rolling for the Hips and Glutes:

- Sit on the foam roller and roll back and forth to release tension in the glutes and hips.

8. Massage Ball Release for the Neck:

- Lie on your back with a massage ball under your neck.

- Gently move your head from side to side to release tension in the neck fascia.

Cool-down:

- Finish the routine with 5-10 minutes of gentle stretching, focusing on areas that have been targeted in the routine.

Notes:

- Perform each exercise slowly and mindfully, paying attention to your body's feedback.

- If you encounter an area of extreme discomfort or pain, reduce the pressure and avoid causing excessive discomfort.

- Customize the routine based on your specific needs and fitness level.

- Consistency is key to experiencing the full benefits of this full-body fascial release routine. Perform it regularly, and over time, you may notice improvements in flexibility and reduced tension in your fascial system.

6.2 Lower Body Fascial Stretching

Lower body fascial stretching is a focused routine designed to enhance flexibility, mobility, and fascial health in the legs, hips, and lower back. This routine is particularly beneficial for individuals seeking to improve lower body flexibility and reduce discomfort. Here's a sample lower body fascial stretching routine:

Equipment Needed: Stretching bands (optional)

Duration: Approximately 15-20 minutes

Warm-up:

- Begin with 5-10 minutes of light aerobic exercise or dynamic stretching to warm up the lower body muscles and increase blood flow.

1. Standing Quadriceps Stretch:

- Stand on one leg and grab your opposite ankle behind you.

- Gently pull your ankle toward your glutes while keeping your knees together.

- Hold for 20-30 seconds on each side.

2. Hamstring Stretch:

- Lie on your back with one leg extended.

- Use a stretching band, if available, to loop around the ball of your extended foot.

- Gently pull the band to stretch your hamstring.

- Hold for 20-30 seconds on each side.

3. Hip Flexor Stretch:

- Kneel on one knee and step your other foot forward.

- Shift your weight forward slightly to stretch the hip flexors.

- Hold for 20-30 seconds on each side.

4. Butterfly Stretch:

- Sit with the soles of your feet touching each other.

- Hold your feet and gently press your knees down toward the floor.

- Hold for 20-30 seconds.

5. Seated Forward Bend:

- Sit with your legs extended in front of you.

- Reach forward to touch your toes or ankles, keeping your back straight.

- Hold for 20-30 seconds.

6. Inner Thigh Stretch:

- Sit with your legs wide apart.

- Gently lean to one side to stretch the inner thigh.

- Hold for 20-30 seconds on each side.

Cool-down:

- Finish the routine with 5-10 minutes of gentle static stretching to relax the lower body muscles.

Notes:

- Focus on deep, mindful breathing during each stretch to enhance relaxation and flexibility.

- Stretch to the point of mild discomfort but not pain. Never force a stretch.

- Customize the routine based on your specific needs and fitness level.

6.3 Upper Body Fascial Sliding

Upper body fascial sliding is a routine that targets the fascial health and flexibility of the upper body, including the shoulders, arms, and neck. This routine emphasizes dynamic movements to promote fascial engagement and overall upper body mobility. Here's a sample upper body fascial sliding routine:

Equipment Needed: None (optional: stretching band for added resistance)

Duration: Approximately 15-20 minutes

Warm-up:

- Begin with 5-10 minutes of light aerobic exercise or dynamic upper body stretches to prepare the upper body for fascial sliding.

1. Arm Circles:

- Stand with your feet shoulder-width apart.

- Extend your arms out to the sides and make large circles

with your arms, forward and then backward.

- Perform 10-15 circles in each direction.

2. Chest Opener:

- Stand tall with your feet hip-width apart.

- Clasp your hands behind your back and gently lift your arms, opening up your chest.

- Hold for 20-30 seconds.

3. Dynamic Shoulder Stretch:

- Stand with your feet hip-width apart.

- Extend your right arm across your body and use your left hand to gently pull your arm closer to your chest.

- Perform this stretch dynamically by moving your arm in and out, feeling the stretch in your shoulder.

- Perform for 20-30 seconds on each arm.

4. Neck Tilt and Rotation:

- Tilt your head to the left and then to the right, feeling the stretch in your neck.

- Perform gentle neck rotations to the left and right, moving your head in a circular motion.

- Hold each stretch for 15-20 seconds.

5. Upper Back Stretch (with stretching band):

- If using a stretching band, hold it in both hands in front of you at shoulder level.

- Gently pull the band apart to stretch your upper back and shoulders.

- Hold for 20-30 seconds.

Cool-down:

- Finish the routine with 5-10 minutes of gentle stretching to relax the upper body muscles.

Notes:

- Pay attention to your body's feedback during each movement and avoid any positions or stretches that cause discomfort or pain.

- Customize the routine based on your specific needs and fitness level.

- Incorporate the use of a stretching band for added resistance if you want to intensify the routine.

CHAPTER 7

Safety and Precautions

7.1 Common Mistakes to Avoid

Fascial exercise is a valuable approach to enhancing flexibility, mobility, and overall well-being, but there are several common mistakes that individuals should avoid to ensure a safe and effective practice:

1. Overexertion: One of the most common mistakes is overexerting oneself. Pushing too hard or attempting advanced fascial exercises without proper preparation can lead to injury or discomfort.

2. Poor Form: Incorrect form can put unnecessary stress on the body and lead to injuries. It's crucial to maintain proper alignment and posture during exercises.

3. Ignoring Pain: Fascial exercise may cause mild discomfort due to the release of tension, but sharp or intense pain should not be ignored. If a stretch or movement is painful, back off and reassess your technique.

4. Lack of Consistency: The benefits of fascial exercise come with regular practice. Inconsistency in your routine may limit the effectiveness of the exercises.

5. Neglecting Warm-up: Skipping a proper warm-up can increase the risk of injury. Always start your fascial exercise routine with light aerobic activity or dynamic stretching to prepare your muscles and fascia.

6. Rushing Movements: Fascial exercise is most effective when performed slowly and mindfully. Rushing through movements can diminish the benefits and increase the risk of injury.

7. Neglecting Hydration: Hydration is crucial for the health of your fascial tissues. Dehydrated fascia can become stiff and less flexible, so remember to stay well-hydrated before, during, and after your fascial exercise routine.

8. Focusing Solely on Flexibility: While improving flexibility is a common goal, neglecting strength and stability training can lead to imbalances in the body. Incorporate strength and stability exercises into your routine for a holistic approach.

9. Comparing Yourself to Others:
Everyone's body is unique, and
progress varies from person to person.
Avoid comparing your progress to
others, as it can lead to frustration or
overexertion.

10. Not Listening to Your Body: It's
essential to listen to your body and
modify exercises as needed. If
something doesn't feel right or causes
pain, adjust your approach or consult
with a professional.

7.2 Precautions for Beginners

If you're new to fascial exercise, there
are several precautions and
considerations to keep in mind to
ensure a safe and enjoyable
experience:

1. Start Slowly: Begin with simple fascial exercise routines and gradually progress to more advanced techniques as you build strength and flexibility.

2. Consult a Professional: Consider working with a certified fascial exercise instructor or physical therapist when starting, especially if you have any existing medical conditions or injuries.

3. Focus on Form: Pay close attention to your form and alignment during exercises to prevent injury and optimize the benefits of fascial exercise.

4. Warm-up: Always perform a proper warm-up to prepare your muscles and fascia for the exercise routine.

5. Listen to Your Body: If an exercise feels painful or

uncomfortable, adjust or stop. It's essential to listen to your body's feedback and avoid pushing too hard.

6. Stay Hydrated: Adequate hydration is crucial for healthy fascial tissue. Ensure you're drinking enough water throughout the day.

7. Rest and Recovery: Allow your body time to recover between fascial exercise sessions. Overtraining can lead to fatigue and injury.

8. Modify for Comfort: If you have limitations, injuries, or medical conditions, modify exercises to suit your needs. Seek guidance from a professional if necessary.

9. Be Patient: Results in fascial exercise may take time. Be patient and consistent in your practice.

7.3 When to Consult a Professional

While fascial exercise can be accessible and safe for many individuals, there are specific situations where consulting a professional is advisable:

1. Existing Medical Conditions: If you have any pre-existing medical conditions, especially those affecting your musculoskeletal system, it's essential to consult with a physical therapist, orthopedic specialist, or other healthcare provider before starting a fascial exercise routine.

2. Recent Injuries: If you've had recent injuries, surgery, or acute conditions, a professional can help you determine when and how to reintroduce fascial exercise safely.

3. Chronic Pain: If you experience chronic pain, it's advisable to seek the guidance of a healthcare provider or physical therapist to create a fascial exercise routine that is both effective and pain-free.

4. Limited Mobility: If you have limited mobility or severe joint issues, working with a professional can help you adapt exercises to your unique needs.

5. Performance Enhancement: Athletes looking to optimize their performance through fascial exercise may benefit from working with a specialized trainer or coach who understands the specific demands of their sport.

6. Customized Programs: If you're looking for a customized fascial exercise program tailored to your goals, body type, and abilities, a professional instructor or therapist can provide the best guidance.

Consulting a professional is particularly important when dealing with medical conditions, injuries, or unique performance goals. They can provide personalized guidance and ensure that your fascial exercise routine aligns with your individual needs and objectives.

CHAPTER 8

Integrating Fascial Exercise into Your Fitness Routine

8.1 Combining Fascial Exercise with Strength Training

Integrating fascial exercise with strength training is a powerful way to promote overall fitness, improve functional movement, and optimize the health of your fascial system. Here's how you can effectively combine these two forms of exercise:

1. Warm-Up: Begin your workout with a brief fascial exercise routine to prepare your body. Focus on foam rolling or dynamic stretching to loosen fascial tissue and improve mobility.

2. Dynamic Stretching: Incorporate dynamic stretching exercises as part of your warm-up or between strength training sets. Dynamic stretches engage the fascial system and help improve flexibility while promoting blood flow.

3. Fascial Strengthening: Some strength training exercises naturally engage the fascial system, particularly those that involve functional, multi-planar movements. Examples include kettlebell swings, medicine ball exercises, and resistance band exercises.

4. Post-Workout Fascial Release: After your strength training session, dedicate time to fascial release techniques. Use foam rollers or massage balls to target areas of tension and prevent fascial adhesions from forming.

5. Variety of Movements: Ensure that your strength training routine includes a variety of movements that challenge different muscle groups and fascial lines. This variety promotes fascial health and overall body balance.

6. Mindful Movements: Approach both strength training and fascial exercise with mindfulness. Pay attention to your body's feedback and use proper form in all exercises to prevent injury and maximize benefits.

8.2 Incorporating Fascial Exercise into Yoga and Pilates

Fascial exercise can complement yoga and Pilates by adding a dimension of myofascial release, enhanced mobility, and holistic wellness. Here's how to incorporate fascial exercise into your yoga and Pilates practice:

1. Pre-Yoga/Pilates Warm-Up: Begin your yoga or Pilates session with a brief fascial exercise warm-up. Foam rolling or massage ball release can help prepare your body for the mindful movement ahead.

2. Fascial Stretching: Integrate fascial stretching into your yoga or Pilates routine. Incorporate dynamic stretches or yoga poses that emphasize the fascia's role in movement. Examples include cat-cow poses, supine leg stretches, or modified sun salutations.

3. Fascial Release in Restorative Poses: Incorporate fascial release techniques in restorative or yin yoga poses. Use props like foam rollers and massage balls to release tension during passive stretches and poses.

4. Awareness of Fascia: Develop a greater awareness of the fascia during your practice. Mindfully engage your fascial system by focusing on the connections between different body parts and the myofascial lines that run through the body.

5. Integration of Breath: Coordinate your breath with fascial exercise during your yoga or Pilates practice. Mindful breathing enhances the mind-body connection and supports fascial release.

6. Cool-Down and Fascial Release:
After your yoga or Pilates session,
incorporate post-workout fascial
release techniques. Target areas that
have been engaged during the
practice, like the hips, shoulders, and
back.

7. Consistency: Regularly integrate
fascial exercise into your yoga or
Pilates routine to experience the
cumulative benefits of enhanced
flexibility, mobility, and holistic
wellness.

8.3 Embracing a Holistic Approach to Health and Wellness

Fascial exercise naturally aligns with
a holistic approach to health and
wellness, as it acknowledges the

interconnectedness of the body and mind. Here's how to embrace this holistic perspective:

1. Mind-Body Connection: Develop a strong mind-body connection through fascial exercise. Pay attention to physical sensations, emotions, and energy levels during your practice. This awareness promotes holistic well-being.

2. Breath Awareness: Emphasize the role of breath in fascial exercise. Breath awareness fosters relaxation, reduces stress, and supports a deeper mind-body connection.

3. Nutritional Support: Complement your fascial exercise routine with a balanced diet that nourishes the fascial tissues. Proper nutrition supports fascial health and overall wellness.

4. Hydration: Stay well-hydrated to maintain the health and pliability of fascia. Adequate hydration ensures that the fascial tissues remain supple and flexible.

5. Sleep and Recovery: Prioritize quality sleep and recovery. Adequate rest is essential for the body's repair and rejuvenation processes, which include fascial health.

6. Emotional Well-Being: Recognize the emotional aspects of fascial health. Emotional stress and tension can affect the fascial system, so practices like meditation and stress management can contribute to holistic wellness.

7. Professional Guidance: Seek the guidance of healthcare professionals, fitness instructors, and therapists who understand the holistic approach to health and can support you in your fascial exercise journey.

8. Personalized Approach:

Understand that your holistic wellness journey is unique. Customize your approach to fascial exercise, nutrition, and wellness to fit your individual needs and goals.

Integrating fascial exercise into your fitness routine while embracing a holistic approach to health, you can experience the profound benefits of improved flexibility, reduced discomfort, enhanced mobility, and a deeper sense of overall well-being.